21 Days

To
Ultimate
Health and Wellness

21 DAYS

TO
ULTIMATE
HEALTH AND WELLNESS

Marques,
Prosperity, Abundance, and Wealth
is yours now!
Peace and Be More
Coach E

ERICH C. NALL 4·16·11

TAKAMA PUBLISHING HOUSE
CALIFORNIA

Published and distributed by:
TAKAMA Publishing House
Gardena, California 90249

Cover Design: Quillard, Inc.

Formatting: Alpha Enterprises

First Printing, January 2011
10 9 8 7 6 5 4 3 2 1

1. Self Help (New Age) 2. Health & Fitness: General 3. Family &
   Relationship: Health

ISBN: 978-0-9831850-0-0

TAKAMA Publishing House
14752 Crenshaw Blvd. Ste. 350
Gardena, California 90249
(310) 859-5526

Website: www. ultimatetransformations.com
E-mail: info@ultimatetransformations.com

DEDICATION

This book is dedicated to my loving family and friends, who have all impacted my life. I strive to do my best and be my best in everything, and I thank you all for the unconditional love.

My special dedication is to four beautiful ladies, my wife and three daughters. They make every moment in my life special.

TABLE OF CONTENTS

FOREWORD

What is Ultimate Transformation? Is it the before and after – the promise of a skinny, smiling new you with a tape measure around your waist and the man or woman of your dreams on your arm? Is it a surgically enhanced self that is ageless and perfect and ready for prime time? Is it the kinder, gentler you who has, through meditation or medication found a way to smooth out those emotional wrinkles and portray a pleasantly serene blandness all day every day? Does the idea of Ultimate Transformation imply, as do so many television commercials, movies and videos, that there is something *wrong* with the current you that requires immediate alteration? The answer to all of these questions is a resounding – *no!*

While most of us have things about ourselves we would like to change, or strive to master, the basic concept of Ultimate Transformations is about falling in love with you! It is not about turning yourself into a carbon copy of someone else, or fixing you because you are broken. It is about finding your true essence, distilling, bolstering, and honoring it. Ultimate Transformations is about *falling in love with the highest image of yourself.*

Erich Nall and his team begin with the assumption that, at their essence, all people are good. It is an orientation that changes the game. Instead of shaming, bullying, disciplining or bribing us to be our best, we are given the tools to improve and gain the mastery we desire. We are then encouraged to make a commitment to ourselves, for ourselves, and in our own best interest. With this foundation, we are able to share this mastery with our families and community without guilt, shame, or strain and this sharing becomes the natural effect of our leading by example.

I stumbled across Ultimate Transformations Training on my journey back to wellness following the birth of my son. Walking in a beautiful Los Angeles park one day, I heard the voice in my head say "Why are you walking? You are a runner," and at that moment, I took off running after three years of not working out at all. Months later, I met Erich Nall when he made a casual remark about my running gait. I then realized that I had been working out injured without really noticing, or maybe, I just put the pain in the vast "you're not as young as you used to be" category and assumed it was supposed to hurt to run at my age!

Observing his cheerful (and amazingly fit) group of men and women, professional athletes and amateurs, I decided to give the workout a try. As a fitness enthusiast, I have sampled many trainers, systems, disciplines and fads over the years and some have worked well for me. I have always believed you should engage in whatever fitness regimen you will actually show up and DO. As a happy "self-help-a-holic," I have benefited from the books and teachings of people like Marianne Williamson, Iyanla Vanzant and Deepak Chopra. As a radio and television broadcaster and activist I have always enjoyed seeking new knowledge to stay informed, engaged and engaging on the mental level. Never had I found a place where all three aspects of my training consciously intersect, until Ultimate Transformations.

Erich Nall has created a system in Ultimate Transformations Training where fitness is defined as the holistic health of mind, body and spirit. He has invented a space where life coaching, fitness training and spiritual development take place in the same arena. It is a concept that seems so natural, even obvious, yet it is unique, and it makes all the difference in the world. With the physical affirming the spiritual, the spiritual uplifting the mental and so on, I am able to fully integrate the goals for my mind, body and spirit for the first time. With my busy schedule and demanding lifestyle, as a working mother with a young child, putting all of these puzzle pieces together in one place (with only one spot on the schedule!) is important. It means I never have to feel like I am choosing one important aspect of myself over the other while leaving a part neglected.

Erich Nall embodies his own system. He is a gifted and intuitive life coach. He is a fitness trainer and an athletic coach who is deeply rooted in the science of physiology and nutritional principals. He is an athlete. He is also an MBA whose successful academic career created in him a lifelong scholar and teacher. Thus Erich is able to lead by example even as he teaches us to do so. His incredible commitment to ongoing mastery of physical, mental, and spiritual wellness gives him the credibility and unique perspective to bring forth an Ultimate Transformation. This transformation, which is truly a process of transcendence from the self to the higher self, is empowering for not only the individual, but, the families and the communities they touch.

The empowerment is contagious! I have noticed it spreading to other aspects of my life. Ultimate Transformations is not just a training regimen, it is a set of tools and a system for forming and/or breaking habits. As such, it applies to all goals, from my work life to my personal relationships. Because Ultimate Transformations equips each of us with these tools and teaches us the system. Nall is truly teaching us to fish, rather than handing us that tasty plate of fried (or baked) red snapper!

Needless to say, it no longer hurts when I run. I have thrown the notion of, "you're not as young as you used to be" into the trash bin! Additionally, I am enjoying the fact that as I have entered the notorious "over 40" category, I look and feel better than I did ten years ago.

Of course, I am not "there" yet, and in fact my "there" is constantly shifting these days. As I reach one goal, I now recalibrate for the next cycle. Erich says "there is no before and after – there is only right now," and right now, I am busy *falling in love with the highest image of myself!* I am truly grateful to be Ultimately Transformed...

Dominique DiPrima, Radio Host & Producer
December 1, 2010

What People Are Saying:

"Coach E hasn't been just a trainer to me. He's been a listening ear, a positive role model, a husband and father (role) model, and a constant motivator. He has taught me what real commitment is. There is no "run around" with Coach E. He makes the boys grow into men, and then those men can make other boys into men. Coach E is transparent and positively contagious."

-Brandon Hampton – Corner back, Detroit Lions

~

"As a healthcare professional, I know how to work out. I came to Coach E because I was bored with my workout and needed motivation. What I received in return was so much more than I expected. Coach E motivated and inspired my mind, body and spirit, which helped me become a better person for myself, my family and for my patients. Thank you Coach E. Knowing you has truly been a blessing."

- Dr. Dionne McClain, CEO, McClain Sports & Wellness, Clinical Professor, USCHS

~

"...I first met Erich when my son was 16 years old while looking for someone that could help Alterraun with his speed. One of the best things that happened in our lives was meeting and working with Erich and Ultimate Transformations. Ultimate Transformations played a key role in my son's success. Ultimate Transformations helped my son develop his body and mind, and become an outstanding athlete. Thanks again Erich."

- Robert Verner, father of the Tennessee Titans corner-back Alterraun Verner

~

"E is more than a physical trainer; he is a friend, mentor & someone I admire. As a child, he installed a work ethic in me that I have till this day. As a person with a speech impediment,

he helped me to gain confidence & told me to always believe in myself. Congrats coach E!"
  - *Corey Long, South Gate Middle School teacher, real estate agent.*

~

"Coach E can get you moving from zero to fifty RPM's at any age!"
  - *Yvonne A. Scott, District Student Information System Computer Technician at Inglewood Unified School District.*

~

"Coach E knew how to design a work out and food plan to fit my needs exactly! I wanted to keep my behind, a slim waist with a six pack and everything else trim and lean, and he did exactly that!"
  - *SACHA KEMP, actress/model*

~

"Before my 50th birthday, my goal was to lose weight and get in shape. I was introduced to Coach E and with his mind and body workout, I was able to reach my goal within 6 months. Thanks Coach E for my ultimate transformation."
  -*Karen Paysinger, Intervention Support Coordinator, Crescent Heights Elem.*

~

It's been said that there are two important days in a man's life. First, the day he was born. Second, the day he found out why he was born. As the founder of the nationally recognized Black Barbershop Health Outreach Program, I am often reminded of the day my purpose and assignment was distilled and refined. It happened one morning after a workout with Coach E.

This was no ordinary morning. I was consumed by a heavy emotional weight that he easily recognized. The timing of his words was pivotal. Go and help somebody he said. The thought of helping someone else when I was going through this difficult time was not in my immediate consciousness. I was hurting and I was hurting bad. This experience culminated into a personal transformation.

The Black Barbershop Health Outreach Program was born whereas we screen men for diabetes and high blood pressure in barbershops around the country. To date, we have screened over 25,000 men in over 26 cities. The Mind, Body and Spiritual elements of the Ultimate Transformation Program were fundamental in the preparation to fulfill my life's purpose."
- Dr. Bill J. Releford, D.P.M.
Founder, DAP Foundation /
Black Barbershop Health Outreach Program
Associate Professor

~

"Over our five year relationship, Coach E has been an incredible force in my life, but more importantly the time he has invested training my teenage son, both mentally and physically has truly been immeasurable."
- David Plummer III, VP of Sales

~

I have never worked harder or laughed harder during a workout than I did when training with Erich Nall. His eye for technique and relentless belief transformed my beach volleyball game and enabled me to make the necessary changes to lead the Pro Tour in digs per game in 2007. Not only is Erich the best at what he does, he is also a visionary. He has created a fitness and sports environment where people come together. A training session with Erich may have everyone from Olympic athletes, Hollywood celebrities, inner city kids, housewives, and weekend-warrior athletes improving their lives through a personalized fitness program. He's created an amazing environment that feels like family, and brings out the best in everyone he works with. Thank you Erich.
- Jen Pavley, Pro Beach Volleyball Athlete

~

7

"At the very core of any necessary change, three relevant areas must be engaged for a successful outcome: body, mind and spirit. Erich has been able to include these key components into his work as a trainer, mentor and teacher thereby producing profound results. My time spent with "Coach E" has been nothing short of transformational."
- *Valezra Earl, Human Resources & Administration Manager*

~~~

PREFACE

For over twenty years, I have been involved in health and wellness. Initially, as the founder of a tutorial program for youth, ages 7 to 18, then as a strength, speed and conditioning coach and personal trainer. I work with individuals and consistently assist them in making the necessary changes in their lives to reach tremendous heights. Successes range from a youth overcoming extreme odds to make their way into college then graduation, to college students beating the odds, working hard and achieving the goal of playing professional sports. I work with everyday people, to help them lose incredible amounts of weight, that go on to run marathons, as well as individuals with dreams of stardom, who train hard to get their body and mind right and then go on to make a name in Hollywood.

All of these instances show how a person can have a desire, choose something in life, make a commitment to the desire, then go on to reap the benefits of success according to their own definition of success.

I have written 21 Days to Ultimate Health and Wellness, because through all of these years of being a support to hundreds of individuals, I realize that I have been walking my clients, family and friends through a formula that allows them to reach their goals in health and in life. The process has been the same regardless of whether the goals are in education, health, athletics, or wealth building. I have used

9

the same process to concentrate my own focus to finish this book.

The process begins with a choice and requires your belief and commitment. For many it has taken several decades to form the bad habits that exist as deterrents in their current lives. However, you can take the first steps to your Ultimate Transformation. Spend 21 days on your journey to Ultimate Health and Wellness. Is the life you desire worth 21 days of commitment? I believe it is.

INTRODUCTION

THE ULTIMATE TRANSFORMATION WAY TO HEALTH AND WELLNESS

You have chosen this book because you are looking for a system that will help you achieve mental, physical and spiritual wellness. Ultimate Transformations Training is that system. The Ultimate Transformations Training way has it's base in physical fitness. However, it focuses on the whole individual: the individual who is striving for Mental, Physical and Spiritual Mastery. Simply put, every facet of your mind, your body and your soul must be engaged in this system and the techniques that are outlined herein, for complete transformation.

Your goal is to experience life from a place of true health and wellness. To do so, you must place focused emphasis on all three fundamental components: Mental, Physical and Spiritual. When we seek to get the most out of our individual lives, maximum/**ULTIMATE** effort must be put forth in order to achieve maximum results. If any of the three areas within is not in line with what you want, know that you have the power to do something about it. You can change the way you see yourself in any, or in all, of these areas. When you learn to see yourself and the world around you positively, you **TRANSFORM**. Finally, to continue to experience the maximum and most positive change in yourself and your life, you must have a clear and definitive goal as well as a plan to achieve it. You must be willing to get up everyday with the goal and your plan in mind. You will execute the details of the plan by **TRAINING**. The formula for this foundation is found in Ultimate Transformations Training.

Everything that occurs in your life, either in your family, your community or your work, has its origin in your individual self. This is evident in the way you react to the various situations that are presented. Whether situations are positive or negative, you possess a power within that allows you to elevate yourself above it. The power is in your CHOICE. You can change any and everything about yourself simply by making a new choice that puts you in direct alignment with the new direction you want to pursue.

Sometimes, current situations can seem very overwhelming and almost impossible to overcome. In today's society, the media spends a great deal of time bombarding the airwaves with stories of financial ruin, high unemployment, declining educational facilities and the lack of opportunities for our children. The daily news stories reflect a youth generation that seems to be lost and out of control. The family is being portrayed as an institution that appears to be crumbling. The health of the world is shown to be on a steady decline as obesity in youth and adults continues to increase. The media supplies us with one negative story after another. Do not be discouraged. Do not fall prey to all of this negative energy. Stop for a moment and take a look around. Evaluate yourself inside and out. After taking some time to assess your situation, begin to focus on your belief in all that is good. And, if you believe as I do, that there is something that you can do personally to help you be better and feel better, well, do something! Right now, in this moment, you can choose differently. You can make the next choice that is in alignment with whatever it is that you want. The power in choosing does not stop there. Think positively about yourself and your surroundings. Believe in yourself. Believe that you can accomplish anything. Do something. *Don't just talk about it, be about it!*

Know that your journey may have some challenges, but with consistent effort, you will *always* prevail. You must get started, and never, ever, give up! No matter what the situation, or dilemma, you can only start where you are now. Take your first step. Take it!

You are now ready to begin Ultimate Transformations Training's, *21 Days to Ultimate Health and Wellness*. This book helps you understand that the greatness that you are born with is the key to achieving any goal that you set. When you demonstrate greatness through your achievements, it can influence your family, your community, and ultimately the world. Use the concepts in this book as a guide and a reference. Feel free to use these concepts in every phase of your life. Know that you are a Divine Creation that has been brought to earth to feel, do and experience greatness in all aspects of your life. You are more than your mind. You are more than your body. You are more than your soul. The true you, is comprised of all three of these powerful components. You were born great, and this life is about letting your greatness shine. Let Ultimate Transformations Training help you find the way!

Peace and be more!

Erich C. Nall (Coach E)

THE
FOUNDATION

Chapter 1

The Roadmap to Ultimate Transformation

Health and Wellness Is Your Choice

You have selected this book to read, which indicates that you have a true interest in your personal health and wellness. You also have the desire to improve your personal health and wellness and are ready to work for this change. If these statements are true, then I advise you to continue reading!

Your health and wellness are the most important components to your individual success. In contrast, let's take a look at a machine for a moment. Note that a machine that does not work properly, or is not operating at peak efficiency, would be considered defective. A defective machine will most always produce a sub-par product, if it produces anything at all. A defective machine is incapable of producing a high-quality product. Now, let's consider the body. The body is the most intricate *machine* in all of creation. In this moment, ask yourself the following questions: "Do I produce a sub-par product?" "Can I be more efficient?" If the answer to either of these questions is yes, then, let's continue.

What is Health and Wellness?

When the focus is on health and wellness, an individual devotes equal attention and effort to improving their mental, spiritual and physical wellbeing. Mentally, you may focus on education and the ability to choose. Spiritually, the focus may be placed on acting from a position of complete belief, while the Physical focus may be on your day-to-day action or activity.

When your health and wellness is a priority, all three components of self, Mental, Spiritual and Physical, are given equal attention. From this point, the creation of the individual self that has the ability to meet the everyday challenges *begins*. More significantly, with improved health and wellness you begin to operate, from a place that is more inner driven because there will be greater clarity in your thinking. You become more innovative and creative, thus bringing you closer to achieving greater objectives individually. This allows you to affect your surroundings in a much more positive way. Personal health and wellness is the foundation to gaining the confidence to pursue greater achievements and the willingness to act outside of the status quo. These are the rudimentary qualities that advance society to greater heights.

Yes, the world can change for the better, beginning with you! In his book *As A Man Thinketh*, James Allen writes "Circumstances do not make the man, but will reveal himself to himself." This statement indicates that when you take this moment to evaluate who you are in every aspect of your individual life, you will see that your physical or mental (character), whether it is good/positive or bad/negative, is the culmination of your previous thoughts and habits. These thoughts and habits are revealing themselves in your present life. Conversely, if you are not satisfied with an aspect of your present self, you can change it simply by changing how you think in regard to the particular aspect. This also means that you possess a tremendous power that you carry inside of your individual self. Remember, you cannot express powers that you do not possess. The only way by which you may secure possession of power is to become conscious (aware) of power, and you never become conscious (aware) of power until you learn that all power resides within. Your power lies within you, RIGHT NOW!

This power that we all possess can be used to control how we think TODAY! How and what we think controls our actions. This should bring you excitement over the limitless possibilities that you have to experience the life that you desire. Right now is the time for action. Don't wait. The longer you delay, the longer it will take you to experience the incredible life that you long to have. That new life starts with your individual health and wellness. Where do you begin? Your starting place is right where you are, in this current moment. The journey to the new you and a new life begins with a single step. Take it! Congratulations, you have just begun your Ultimate Transformation!

The Foundation to Choice

There are three components that must be understood, before we discuss your innate ability to choose for yourself, with your highest potential in mind. These components are: human potential, control of self, and the All Good. I refer to these three components as "characteristics to better choosing." First, human potential refers to the knowledge that all human potential is unlimited. Second, self-control is based on the fact that the only thing that an individual can control is his or her own action. Third, All Good, refers to the belief that the true nature of all God's creations is good. While the following chapters will expand on these characteristics, let me briefly introduce the concepts here.

The first Characteristic that we all possess is an unlimited human potential. Whatever you, as an individual, choose to become, do, or believe, you must consider it done. All that is sought after, is available now, and will manifest itself. The requirement is a clear and focused mind, to allow the thoughts and the full belief in the thoughts, to become one. Thought is the origin of all creation. Human potential can only be limited by your thoughts. The thought/ belief that you carry about yourself, your family, community, or environment, is the only limiting factor in the ultimate flourishing of each of these areas.

The second Characteristic that we all possess is control over ourselves. You cannot dictate the actions of another, and conversely, no one can dictate the actions you choose to take. The only control another can have over you is the control that you give to them. Focus on self, and the actions that you are choosing.

The third Characteristic that we all possess is belief in the knowledge that the basic nature of all living things is good. You must know and believe this fact so deeply that it becomes second nature. Because from this belief comes the understanding that as an individual, you are good, and what will come to you will be good. Specifically stated, everyone's basic true nature is good (God).

Goal Identification – *Fall in love*

To achieve anything of substance in your individual life, you must have clear goals and objectives as well as a plan to reach your desired outcome. When you choose specific goals and objectives that are based on your own personal happiness, you must use positive thought and take positive actions towards your objective everyday, no matter how small the step. Each action puts you closer to your goal. Creating a specific action plan ensures that your actions are leading you in the direction of your desired destination. This book will help you to develop your individual action plan, based on your own thoughts, choices, and habits. My personal goal is to help you *fall in love with the highest image of yourself.*

To fall in love with the highest image of yourself, two definitive actions must occur. First, you must create the highest and best image of yourself by defining who you are in all aspects of your life. Second, you must make a choice as to how you view your individual self. Choice is a power that is with you in every moment of your day, every day of your life. Choice is the right, power, or chance, to choose an option. Choice means that there is an abundance and a variety from which to choose. You have the power to choose the best and most preferred part of every-thing. The ability to choose carries a great deal of power and all of us have access to that power, because it comes from within.

Let's contemplate this internal power for a moment. Understand that you have the power to choose, any characteristic, any career, or, the person you would like to become. This will be the starting point to creating the image of yourself with which you *choose* to fall in love.

Habits

With the power to choose in mind, there is serious and determined work that must be done. It is time to take action. We have established that we are the culmination of all our previous thoughts. The prerequisite to action is thought and it is with this acknowledgement that we execute the power to choose.

You must choose to create the highest image of self that possesses everything that you desire. This highest self is the image that we must choose to fall in love with. Now, how to proceed? How do you move forward from this point of conception to develop and execute your plan? Make progress by replacing your old thoughts and habits with new self-elevating thoughts and habits. Yes, I use the term habit because your habits are your repeated actions. Almost every-thing that you do in a day is the result of habit. Habits are conditioned responses formed from doing an action repeatedly. When habits are formed, you don't have to think about them. Little thought is given to actions that have become habits, and you are not consciously aware of many of these actions. The journey to change these habits may present a bit of a challenge. Habits can be both positive and negative forces in your life. If you become aware of a habit that does not produce positive results in your life, you must find the strength and determination to replace it. The old negative habits are to be replaced with new positive actions that are consistent with the desired life you want to live.

Current habits are the result of how you have previously thought of yourself and your surroundings. If your thoughts are not in alignment with your desires, your actions will lead you even further from your objectives. You want to change any habits that are contrary to your true potential.

All that we can imagine doing and all that we will do, or fail to do, is a result of the picture of "self," that we carry. That picture is derived from the sum total of our experiences from birth to the present day. This picture becomes the basis of all your behavioral patterns. With this understanding, one can see the need for a Roadmap to Ultimate Transformation.

The following exercise is designed to help you begin to gain an initial perspective of self, at this very moment. After completing this book and the exercises that follow, you will be asked to repeat this exercise:

PICTURE OF SELF – SNAPSHOT #1

DATE: _____

HOW DO I FEEL ABOUT MYSELF TODAY?

MENTALLY? _____

_____

_____

_____

_____

PHYSICALLY? _____

_____

_____

_____

_____

SPIRITUALLY? _____

_____

_____

_____

_____

_____

WHERE DO I SEE MYSELF IN THE NEXT 12 MONTHS

_____
_____
_____
_____
_____

WHERE DO I SEE MYSELF IN THE NEXT 24 MONTHS?

_____
_____
_____
_____
_____

WHERE DO I SEE MYSELF IN THE NEXT 5 YEARS?

_____
_____
_____
_____
_____

AM I CHOOSING TO DO THE WORK TO CHANGE?

[ ] YES, BECAUSE _____
_____
_____
_____
_____

I ask you, "Are you ready for true health and wellness?" This is not a quick fix program. It is a lifestyle change, a lifestyle change that requires your time and commitment. I am asking you to make the best investment that you can ever make in your life.

INVEST IN YOUR OWN PERSONAL HEALTH AND WELLNESS

CHAPTER 2

HUMAN POTENTIAL

Ask yourself, how do I think? Do I believe that if I choose something in my life I can obtain it? Every human being, wherever you are right now, is the combined result of all previous thoughts. One of my favorite lines of all books, *As A Man Thinketh*, by James Allen, states, "Circumstances do not make the man but they will reveal himself to himself." Simply put, this means that how you react to situations is based on how you thought prior to those situations. For example, a bank robber doesn't just wake up one day and say he's going to rob a bank. He has thought about robbing banks and then the opportunity makes itself available and he robs the bank.

When looking at your human potential, if you believe that regardless of the obstacle, the situation

no matter what the circumstance, that you will benefit, you will become better, you will become stronger,
then you will find a higher level of existence and
these positive outcomes will be the result. To be
more, and to access this human potential, requires
understanding that you have the potential and that
the only limiting factor is your thought. To *be more*,
you must also *believe* in the positive thoughts that
you have. A perfect example of this is seeing our inner city communities where poverty is widespread.
Well, most people in these areas believe more nega-
tively than they do positively, in regards to how and
why the area is poverty-stricken. Unfortunately, as the
negative thinking prevails, the area may continue to
spiral with negative ramifications. Imagine what the
force of positive thinking and action of an entire
neighborhood could do. Would the environment begin to improve? I believe so.

I want you to know that right now you can have
whatever you want and whatever you decide to become is your choice. Your purpose is *your* purpose.
Your purpose is not written in the sky, it is written
in your heart. Through what you believe and what
you choose, you dictate the fulfillment of your purpose. Then once you identify it, you have to commune with your *self* and be willing to make the
choices that move you in the direction that your
heart takes you.

To understand human potential just look around.
You can see human potential and its results as far as
the eye can see. Look at the car that you drive. Look
at the house that you live in. Maybe look at the

boats in the Marina or simply, look at your toaster or, your refrigerator. All of these things were thoughts first and these thoughts came to people, to individuals, who believed in their potential to create something to benefit mankind. From these thoughts, someone created a prototype that has become the object that you see in use today.

OUR THOUGHTS BECOME THINGS

CHAPTER 3

THE ONLY THING THAT YOU CAN CONTROL IS YOURSELF

What is the meaning of "controlling one's self?" First, understand that the prerequisite to all action is thought. The thoughts that you think in regard to yourself only control you. How you affect mankind positively is through your positive thoughts, which result in the production of your positive actions. Then through the positive actions, which you are creating with thought, you create a positive energy and through that positive energy some of the scientific laws of life come into effect.

One universal law is that you attract into your life that which you are. Newton's law of motion states that every action has an equal and opposite reaction. There are proverbs and karma that suggest what goes around comes around. Basically, what you put out you get back. So, when we understand that the only thing that you can control is yourself, choice plays the most important role in your being able to control your output so that you can more directly affect the result or the input (what you receive). How you execute your choice will determine the benefits you receive in this life.

Before I continue, I want you to fully understand what the human being is. We are all bio-chemically different. Everyone's human body is as unique as a fingerprint. Just as everyone has a different finger-print, every human body is different. This now leads us to understand that the human body is different and there is no one on this earth exactly like you. This also means that the purpose that you have inside of you is equally unique from that of everyone else in the world. The gifts you have to offer to the world are unique to you. Your journey is unique.

Again, you can only control yourself, and because you can only control yourself, what you produce through your acts is unique to the world. That means your journey is different than everyone else's so don't look to compare yourself to anyone else. There is no comparison. You may encounter similar situations but everyone's life experiences are different and what drives every individual is the pursuit of happiness. So, your guide to decision-making and making choices largely depends on how you feel about yourself.

Chapter two reminded us that our human potential is unlimited. Great! Now, how do we incorporate our uniqueness with our unlimited human potential? It begins by always acting from a place of good, a place of happiness with oneself.

Make sure that your choices always feel right to you. You alone can make this decision. If something doesn't feel right, it usually means it is not the right thing for you. Your choices should fit comfortably alongside the things that make you feel good, and make you feel happy. While you are experiencing this good feeling, state a purpose, something that you desire out of this happiness. This now starts to give you direction in your life and life choices. You want to continue to make choices that feel right, that also help you reach or obtain what you've identified as your purpose. However, all of these decisions will be based on the knowledge that you alone possess. This is your unique point of view, and it is limitless.

Knowledge comes from experience or education. The word education comes from the Latin word edu-care. Educare means to bring up, bring out, or teach. But for each one of us to be educated, we must move from the unique place inside of us. This statement means that our education comes from understanding that we have everything in our human vessels that we need to be successful. We do not have to use someone else's description of ourselves to define who we are. We define ourselves through what we feel is right, what feels good, and leads us to the obtainment of whatever purpose we have decided to choose. This good feeling must come from a control of self that has been mastered. You control your thoughts.

YOU EFFECT ALL THINGS POSITIVELY OR NEGATIVELY

CHAPTER 4

THE TRUE NATURE OF
ALL CREATION IS GOOD

You are good. You are GREAT! Your true nature is good, and we should expect good out of ALL of our experiences in this life. We have a tendency to believe more strongly that we can't have or can't achieve. The fact is that we CAN, simply based upon the knowledge that our creator created us out of sheer love. This love is the divine power source that is embedded in all of us. When we recognize the fundamental fact that we are all fundamentally good, i.e., our basic nature is good and everyone walking around in this world has the same core essence of goodness, then we begin to recognize the goodness in all that we see.

We are connected to each other by this intrinsic goodness, and this is how our beautiful universe has been formed. The same power that has brought me into existence has brought you into existence has also brought all creation into existence out of the same goodness. With this understanding, we begin to expect good and believe that good is available for us. There is nothing that can stop us from the goodness that is our birthright, but ourselves.

As we recognize the good in all, we can then begin to choose good for ourselves. Since we are in control of ourselves, we have the potential to bring good into our lives. This life that we live is about the manifestation of good. In other words, we are to do good things. As we continue to focus our thoughts upon good things, expect good things, and do good things for others, good things come to us. We produce better relationships. We create businesses that are positive in the community. The world improves because we realize in our own day-to-day activities, there is a higher level of living that we can execute everyday with our choice to do good for ourselves and for others. The cycle that's created through the mindset of good is a better world. Now that we know that we have unlimited potential, we can only control ourselves, and we live with an expectation of good, we have in place the foundation for our next step.

THE GOOD WITHIN
YOU, SURROUNDS YOU

CHAPTER 5

FALL IN LOVE WITH THE
HIGHEST IMAGE OF YOURSELF

Understanding the three core concepts: Human Potential, Control of Self, The True Nature of all creation is Good, is very important. This is the foundation of Ultimate Transformations Training and the process that I'm going to take you through. This process will help you realize the ultimate objective that I want you to have, and that is to *fall in love with the highest image of self.*

With all three of the core concepts, there is an underlying premise that is most important. The underlying premise being that it is your thoughts combined with your beliefs that are the precursors to all actions. Thoughts are things. So, if you continue to think upon whatever situation it may be, it becomes a dominant thought and dominant thoughts become beliefs. And through these beliefs you take actions that are in accordance with what your thoughts are. These actions combined with the dominant and consistent belief in the thoughts cause your actions to become habitual. They are now your habits. So the habits that you have today are the result of the dominant thoughts you've had previously.

You have to understand where your habits come from because if you are going to fall in love with the highest image of yourself, then you have to create the image that is parallel to the *new* thoughts, which will eventually become new beliefs. The new belief will produce different actions, which are new habits. The process that we're about to embark on is about taking older habits and replacing them with new habits, based upon new thoughts, which we believe in, which can then become new actions.

We create these new habits simply by creating your story. To create your story, you're going to have to sit and commune with yourself. That means sit quietly and ask yourself several questions. Ask yourself questions, such as, what is the nature of better health? What is the true nature of perfect health? How can I be pounds lighter? How can I run a marathon? How can I start my own business? What is the nature of starting my own business? To do this you must sit still. Take time out of your day, sit quietly and ask yourself the right questions and make a list. Make a list of items that you may desire. It could be material. I want a new car. I want to lose 20 pounds. I want to run a marathon. I just want to be healthy. I want to be without diabetes. I want to be without hypertension. It could even be all of these things and many more, because human potential is unlimited, and the universe gives us what we contemplate most. It responds directly to our dominant thoughts.

When you begin to ask yourself a series of questions, you'll come up with a list of things to help you create your story. In this story you will write your new you. For example: this new you is three sizes smaller, is able to run a marathon, or is in a loving relationship. Your story will help you create your new image. It is most helpful to contemplate upon yourself with good in mind, good that the universe, God, wants you to have. Once you make these your dominant thoughts, the universe will start putting things in alignment, in front of you, such as the right exercise program and the right nutrition plan. You'll be able to do the things that will lead you to the result that you've created through writing your story.

Your story will be based on the list of your desires; what *you* desire, not what someone else desires for you. You will create this list in Chapter 8. However, in order to tune out the world's perception of who you are, you have to commune with self. So, if you're a husband, you're not embarking upon this journey for your wife, because your wife told you to. Or, if you're a wife, you're not embarking upon this journey because your husband told you to. You're seeking to commune with yourself based upon your personal choice, and because this will bring you happiness. It will bring you confidence. It will bring you strength. As you get closer to becoming who you want to be, the relationships that you have will do as we said before, duplicate good. What goes around comes around. What you put out you get back. If you're a good person, good things come to you. So, make a simple list of your desires. This list may change daily. It's okay. If you need to wake up everyday and make a new list of your desires, that's fine, as long as you are contemplating on yourself and on your image at the highest level that you can. Fall in love with the highest image of YOU. You're on course to change your environ-ment, change your life, your family, your community, and your world, simply by becoming the best *you* that is possible.

NEW BELIEFS CREATE
THE NEW YOU

CHAPTER 6

AFFIRMATIONS

The 21-day process sounds simple enough, however it takes diligence, focus, and patience. It requires your commitment. One way to help you stay on par and on course is through the use of affirmations. An affirmation is a way of supplanting the existing thoughts in your subconscious with those that are most desirable. You use your conscious mind to transfer thoughts to your subconscious mind. Your subconscious is how your body acts and moves without thought. It's what makes your heartbeat and makes the blood run through your veins. You don't think about your heart beating or the blood running through your brain, or the constant breaths that you take. If you don't believe there's a subconscious, I want you to stop now and hold your breath. See how long you can hold it. Yes, pretty soon, probably well within a minute or so, you're going to gasp for air. Your body knows exactly how to take the oxygen it needs, supply the body with it, and cause you to exhale carbon dioxide. It happens all day, every day and you rarely if ever, think about this process. This is the subconscious mind at work.

All of the habits you have are a part of your subconscious because you do certain things, and you think certain thoughts and they become dominant and automatic. Our natural reactions are based upon what we think dominantly which produces what we do dominantly. These are habits. Affirmations help you begin the day thinking on course, or, in a way that will keep you focused on all that is positive and good. I suggest that you find a few affirmations that remind you of your greatness and your connection with the universe. Use these affirmations throughout the day. Anytime you have a negative thought that is not conducive to reaching a higher level, or greater achievement, or greater expression, I ask that you stop the thought immedia-tely and replace it by restating your affirmation.

Here are a few simple affirmations:

- I love and approve of myself
- God supplies all my needs and desires now
- Perfect health is mine now
- All my endeavors are met with success.
- Prosperity is mine now
- There are only positive resolutions
- I am one with the divine and all that is positive is mine
- Today is a perfect day and I bring positive light to all situations

- I give thanks for all the blessings that are bestowed upon me now
- I am love

Use any affirmation that will replace a negative thought with a positive thought and stay consistent. When you think in terms of yourself, just as in your story, you will supplant any negative thoughts that reside in the subconscious with the new positive story. Instead of expecting a negative event or outcome, learn to expect all things good and positive. So creating a story helps you supplant your subconscious with specific ideas of yourself in your immediate future. Read your story, first thing in the morning, midday, and at night. Everyday when you review your list of desires, (those desires that make up who you are) recite your affirmations. These affirmations, these stories, are what some spiritual teachers call prayer, meditation, communing with the higher you. What you are doing is taking your negative thoughts, which produce negative habits, and replacing them with positive thoughts that help you reach higher levels, and create positive habits. This way, you produce greater actions for greater good in your life.

Now that you are familiar with these concepts, let the process of the 21-day Ultimate Transformation journey lead you toward the health and wellness that you desire and that you deserve.

YOUR WORDS ARE POWERFUL

THE
APPLICATION

CHAPTER 7

THE ULTIMATE TRANSFORMATION PROCESS 21 DAYS

We have reviewed the basic concepts of who we are as individuals, moving and shaking in this time continuum we call life. We have learned that our thoughts produce things and the things that we produce can be positive or negative. We now know that our thoughts create our habits. There's a scientific concept that states if you do anything 21 times in a row, a habit is created. So if you have dedicated 21 days to prayer and meditation, by the 22nd day, you will have taken on the meditation mindset. Meditation starts to become a habit. That means you will begin to practice your meditation as a natural reaction.

The concept for health and wellness that you have now embarked upon during this journey is based on developing habits. You will be replacing old habits with new habits. Your new thoughts will be generating these new habits. Your new thoughts that are more positive reside on a much higher level and will produce good.

Now, the Law of Attraction will further assist you because once you focus on the things that you can control, you begin to think better thoughts about yourself and your actions. This has an immediate positive impact because what you put out, you receive. When your output is improved, you attract better input, which leads to a better you. This cycle of positive thought continues to build on itself, which is reflected in an improved family, improvements in the community, and a better life overall.

At the beginning of this book we talked about spiritual concepts and some things that happen inside the individual. Since your transformation happens inside of you, you must be very, very leery of the things that direct or pull from outside, or outside motivations. You want to be sure that whatever you've chosen as your purpose comes from a place within. That good feeling place. One of the things I want you to move away from is the concept of time-based goals. You may have noticed, at the beginning of every New Year, that people make New Year's resolutions. They say, "I'm gong to lose weight this year." They focus on a time frame that is outside of them such as a twelve-month calendar time frame. Time is a concept that is man-made, because the only concept that we must function through is the concept of this moment. Right now. The moment that we have right now is the only time that we have any control in. Your heart beats every moment and a new moment begins with the next heartbeat. The past heartbeat is gone and a new one is here. Boomp! Another moment. Boomp! Another moment. This is how we must live and how we must choose. I want you to use a 21-day cycle to help create habits, and the cycle begins when *you* begin. The start time is not based on the New Year, or summer, or an upcoming event. The start time is based on this moment. It is based on you taking the initiative to start, regardless of the date in the calendar year. Work with your personal calendar of commitment of 21 days. Do not compare yourself with the neighbors, friends, or family members. You are moving through the choices that you make in life according to your own desires, based upon the commencement of 21 days of your commitment. Now, let's begin.

The 21-day process is comprised of five simple steps:

1) Choice. The first step is to choose, decide, and make a decision. There's power in decision. Take this moment and choose health, better health. You have the power. When you choose, it sets in motion the process of you receiving it. So if you're going to make a commitment health-wise, you're going to go through this process with something very simple like exercise. So, if you have made the choice to exercise, *do something*! Now that you have chosen to exercise, what is your next step?

2) Commitment. To commit means to dedicate thought, which produces action, and belief that you can get it done. Make a pledge to yourself that you're going to do something that benefits you. To make this pledge you must understand your own personal value. That's the place from which you make choices, from your good feeling place. So in the example of exercise, you're going to commit, I'm going to commit to three days a week of 30 to 45 minutes of exercise. That's a great commitment.

3) Belief. The third step is having belief. Faith. Understanding that now you want to exercise. If the objective from the very beginning is that I want to become healthier, I'm going to use the act of exercise to get me towards being healthier. You've now made a commitment to three days a week.

You've got to believe that if you commit to these three days a week, it's going to lead you to better health. As you come to balance an understanding of that, the belief continues to grow. Your commitment grows. You will become more and more secure in the choice that you are making.

4) Action. You've made the choice to exercise. You've made a commitment that you're going to walk three days a week, for example. You believe that walking three days a week will help you meet your goals. This fourth

54

step is to get it done. Take action! You've got to get up and DO IT! So three days a week, you're going to wake up at six in the morning and walk for 45 minutes. You've got to do it. No excuses. You can't give yourself an out. You've got to commit. You execute the commitment by getting it done. Sometimes you don't feel good. Well, let's not make excuses. Perseverance is how you replace the old habit. Get it done through the commitment that you made, three days a week. You do this for, okay you said three days a week, so that means in seven weeks of walking, three days a week (21 workout days), you will have created a habit. That habit of walking three days a week will have gotten you closer to what you've chosen, better health.

5) Evaluation/Recalibration. You feel good about your progress. Now it's time to sit down with the fifth step and evaluate and re-calibrate. You look at yourself and say, "Wow, I got up some days, I didn't feel good and I still made it happen. What I have noticed is that instead of walking two miles in 30 minutes, I walk four miles in 45 minutes. I feel much better." You're making your own personal evaluation. It's not based on anyone else's evaluation, because your evaluation is the only thing that matters. How you feel about yourself is key. You might see a loss of weight. You might see tone in the body. These are all positive things. In this evaluation, you must celebrate your achievements because those achievements will

ERICH C. NALL

spark the next step. That next step is to revisit the place of choos-ing once again.

Now, say you decide, you like walking the 45 minutes. Then, your first commitment is to walking for 45 minutes and when you recalibrate, this may increase to an hour. Concurrently, you decide to commit to improving your nutrition. The process and cycle begin again. You have created the habit of walking. Now you want to create a new nutritional habit focused on eating better. You are building habits that lead you towards your ultimate goal and purpose. This is the process and the cycle that you can use for the rest of your life, in an and all areas you decide.

You are now on your way!

*A JOURNEY BEGINS
WITH A SINGLE STEP*

Chapter 8

Put it on Paper

Goal setting helps to provide the catalyst for change. It is also helpful to see your goals and desires on paper. Before you start to list your desires from a personal happiness place, sit down and commune with yourself. Find a quiet place, where you are comfortable and you won't be interrupted. Quiet your mind by simply focusing on each breath that you take. Inhale then exhale. Relax your body from all tension. Begin by asking yourself personal questions such as, what feels good in health?, how do I see myself physically?, what is the nature of prosperity?, etc. These types of questions help you find the good feeling that directs your desires. All of the questions you ask should give you an answer that feels good to you and only you. Remember the only thing you can control is yourself, so your personal happiness should drive your desires. Take as long as you need to before you begin to make your list of desires. Remember your desires may change daily as you become better at communing with yourself, which is perfectly fine. They may become clearer or more specific.

LIST OF DESIRES

DATE:_____

I DESIRE:

1) _____

2) _____

3) _____

4) _____

5) _____

6) _____

7) _____

8) _____

9) _____

10) _____

List as many or as few desires as you would like.

Additionally, you want to begin each day with the mind-frame or thought origin that is positive and with an expectation of good in your day. You want your thoughts to center around an idea that encompasses your unlimited potential and focuses upon your own specific behavior and GREAT outcomes. Your affirmation can be a simple word or statement, or it may be a lengthy prayer. In any case it must always help you keep your thoughts positive and focused. If your thoughts stray to something negative, release the negative, then return your thoughts to positive. Designate specific times in your day to set aside for affirmations. Morning and night should be mand-atory times to affirm.

AFFIRMATION: CHOOSE YOUR OWN OR SELECT ONE FROM CHAPTER SIX ON AFFIRMATIONS.

_____

_____

_____

_____

_____

_____

_____

_____

_____

_____

_____

21-DAY PROGRAM

CHOOSE: Identify the area in which you feel the need to create a new habit. Make the choice to improve a specific behavior, i.e., eat healthier, practice meditation, etc. Refer to the list of desires that you have listed earlier in this chapter.

I am choosing to: _____

_____

_____

COMMIT: What behavioral change(s) are you going to dedicate thought and action toward. Example: workout 30 minutes of walking, four (4) times per week. You may want to begin with one desired change to begin to master the process:

I am committing to: _____

_____

_____

BELIEVE: Have faith that what you have made a commitment to do, will produce positive results. Affirm your belief in a statement. Example: walking four (4) times per week for 30 minutes is making me healthier by:

_____

_____

_____

DO IT AND LIST IT: You have made the commitment to a choice that you believe in. Now, *get started*! Keep a log of your daily success, based on your commitment. Begin with 21 days. Remember, there are no excuses. List your success each day (within the seven week period).

START DATE: _____

TODAY, MY SUCCESS WAS:	**DATE**
DAY 1 _____	_____
DAY 2 _____	_____
DAY 3 _____	_____
DAY 4 _____	_____
DAY 5 _____	_____

TODAY, MY SUCCESS WAS: DATE

DAY 6 _____ _____

DAY 7 _____ _____

DAY 8 _____ _____

DAY 9 _____ _____

DAY 10 _____ _____

DAY 11 _____ _____

DAY 12 _____ _____

DAY 13 _____ _____

DAY 14 _____ _____

DAY 15 _____ _____

DAY 16 _____ _____

TODAY, MY SUCCESS WAS: <u>DATE</u>

DAY 17 _____ _____

DAY 18 _____ _____

DAY 19 _____ _____

DAY 20 _____ _____

DAY 21 _____ _____

What are you noticing about yourself as your days of success continue to grow? How aware are you of your changing self-image. How are you beginning to grow?

_____

_____

_____

_____

CELEBRATE AND EVALUATE: After meeting your 21-day commitment to your personal change in behavior, celebrate by acknowledging your achievements. List the accomplishments that you've experienced during this time frame.

1) _____ _____

2) _____ _____

3) _____ _____

4) _____ _____

5) _____ _____

RE-CALIBRATE AND CHOOSE: After celebrating your success, re-evaluate your goals based on the progress you have made. Choose the next change in behavior you feel it is time to make. These may be items that you did not focus on in a previous list.

1) _____ _____

2) _____ _____

3) _____ _____

4) _____ _____

5) _____ _____

REPEAT!

Repeat the process: Choose, Commit, Believe, Do it, Celebrate, and Recalibrate. You have now started your own life calendar. A life calendar that is based on your own desires, choices, and change in behavior.

EMBRACE THE PROCESS OF CHANGE

CHAPTER 9

TRANSFORMATIVE NUTRITION

Every subject that we outline and discuss in this book has one underlying premise, and that is you have the power to make decisions for yourself in every aspect of your life. You have the power of choice! This is also a key concept in the area of nutrition.

What is nutrition? Nutrition is the process of providing or obtaining the food necessary for health and growth. This means that the food that you consume should be the most beneficial for your individual health and growth. Food is used for a variety of reasons, including; social gatherings, comfort, an evening out with friends, or a date. As you continue this journey towards self-discovery and learning to expect good in your life, you must begin to look at food primarily for it's nutritional value. Understand that certain foods can enhance your quality of life while others may deteriorate, and cause harm. Your nutrition must come into alignment with your total goal of ultimate health and wellness.

In this process of obtaining ultimate health and wellness, you have come to an understanding that you possess a tremendous power when you choose, and you should make choices with your highest perception of self in mind. Keeping your highest self in mind requires self-mastery in the nutritional area of life.

First, let's take control of our households by getting back to some basic habits. Control, what food you bring into your homes. This means that you have to go out and shop for your own groceries. Shopping for your own groceries means that you will also prepare your own meals. When you shop and prepare our own meals, you are eliminating many variables in your nutrition that you don't have control over. For example, when you eat outside the home (fast food and restaurants), foods are typically prepared with excessive amounts of sodium, sugar, saturated fats and preservatives. These items can turn a potentially healthy meal into an unhealthy one. By preparing your meals you also control and preferably eliminate most harmful ingredients. Providing you with high quality food is not necessarily the objective for fast food restaurants, which is the main reason that it is important to prepare your own meals. Planning and budgeting for meals is generally more financially rewarding as well.

The healthiest eating plan is one that has an emphasis on fruits, vegetables, whole grains, nuts and fat-free or low-fat foods. Additionally, lean meats, preferably poultry and fish, are acceptable. Include beans, (black, red, or white) along with nuts, which are great sources of protein. Beef and pork are considered saturated fats, and should therefore be kept to a minimum. Remember to avoid foods high in saturated trans fats, cholesterol, salt (sodium) and added sugars. Processed foods are canned and packaged foods, which are produced to remain "fresh" on the grocery store shelves. The "processing" of these foods has removed most, if not all, of the nutritional value, and the additives and chemicals make these foods difficult for the body to metabolize.

The second component to the control of your nutrition is portion size. Controlling portion size is required in order to maintain the proper caloric intake. The portion and serving size of your meals will determine your daily caloric intake. There is an optimal number of calories for you to eat each day. This number depends on your age, activity level and whether you're trying to gain, maintain, or lose weight. Even before you know what your daily caloric intake should be, simply changing your mindset during meals to focus on eating in moderation will give you immediate results. By moderation, I am suggesting that you control the portion size of the food or the meal that you consume. In general, the daily average caloric intake for men is 2,550 and for women it is 1,940. This number increases for highly active men and women, and may be slightly lower for those that tend to be less active.

When you super-size meals or fix large portions on the plate, you are setting a personal expectation of over eating without any regard to the actual amount of food required to satisfy your hunger. Your goal is to be able to recognize when you are full and stop eating. If you begin with smaller amounts of food, you may find that you have had enough much sooner than if the plate is filled with two to three times the amount at the start. Being in the habit of eating in moderation will help you to feel that you aren't missing anything. You will also find it easier to maintain control of your caloric intake.

The third nutritional habit is to be sure to drink plenty of water. Water is the body's primary chemical component, comprising an average of 60 percent of your body weight. Every system in your body depends on water. Water flushes toxins out of vital organs, carries nutrients to your cells, and provides a moist environment for ear nose and throat tissue. Water hydrates the body, which in turn helps every function of the body perform better. Water is your daily cleanse. Elimination of waste and toxins is paramount for ultimate health and wellness. Water essentially is the primary component to helping the body eliminate waste and body fat.

As for water consumption guidelines, here is a simple formula; take half your body weight and divide it in half. This is the amount of water in ounces you should ingest in a 24-hour time frame.

Do not gulp the water. It is best to sip the water, drinking no more than 8 ounces in a 30-minute period. Be mindful that when you are exercising regularly you are going to lose quite a lot of water through perspiration. Make sure to drink the required amount, as noted above, plus the amount you lost while exercising. Hydration is very important in your exercise, and it is best to fully hydrate the day before intense workouts. Note that juice, soda, coffee, and alcoholic beverages should not be included when calculating your daily water intake. Make water your staple liquid and you will notice an immediate improvement in your overall health.

The perfect tool to assist you, as you begin to adjust your eating habits, is a daily food log. The food log should detail the time you eat, what you eat and portion size. These three categories will help you see your current nutritional habits and you will be able to make the necessary adjustments to your eating habits that will fit your improved lifestyle.

See Sample Food Log:

ULTIMATE TRANSFORMATIONS
TRAINING
"Mental & Physical Mastery"
Los Angeles, CA

Nutrition Analysis

Name: _____

DATE:				DATE:		
Time	Meal Plan	# Portions		Time	Meal Plan	# Portions
	Breakfast				**Breakfast**	
	Protein -				Protein -	
	Fruit or Grain -				Fruit or Grain -	
	Beverage -				Beverage -	
	Water (oz) -				Water (oz) -	
	Snack				**Snack**	
	Lunch				**Lunch**	
	Protein -				Protein -	
	Vegetable -				Vegetable -	
	Lettuce -				Lettuce -	
	Fruit -				Fruit -	
	Beverage -				Beverage -	
	Misc -				Misc -	
	Water (oz) -				Water (oz) -	
	Snack				**Snack**	
	Dinner				**Dinner**	
	Protein -				Protein -	
	Vegetable -				Vegetable -	
	Lettuce -				Lettuce -	
	Fruit -				Fruit -	
	Beverage -				Beverage -	
	Misc -				Misc -	
	Water (oz) -				Water (oz) -	
	Snack				**Snack**	

THE BODY TEMPLE REQUIRES
YOUR UNDIVIDED ATTENTION

CHAPTER 10

EXERCISE ROUTINES
FOR YOUR
ULTIMATE TRANSFORMATION

Since the focus of this book is on health and wellness, the one component that is the most vital, as well as the most accessible to you, is exercise. You can exercise anywhere, anytime, doing a variety of activities. The key is to get moving, and do something. When total health and wellness is the goal, then the focus cannot be on the mindset alone, nutrition alone, or exercise alone. To achieve total balance, there must be equal concentration placed on all three areas; the mental (thoughts/choice), spiritual (affirmations), and the physical (exercise/nutrition).

Regular physical activity is important for your overall health and fitness. It also helps control body weight by balancing the calories you take in as food with the calories you expend each day. I suggest that you engage in physical activity for at least 30 minutes each day, five days a week. Developing this habit can help you, over time, to increase the intensity of exercise and the duration of your workout.

As you increase the intensity and time that you are physically active, you will experience even greater health benefits. You will control your body weight and lose any excess weight. 60 minutes of exercise, three to five days per week is ideal to prevent weight gain. This regiment combined with low calorie nutrition will foster weight loss, if this is your goal.

For children and teenagers, the program differs slightly. I believe they should be physically active for 60 minutes every day or most every day of the week. Following are three basic workout programs to assist you on your way.

GET ACTIVE NOW!

ULTIMATE BASICS

Prior to commencing any exercise, it is important to begin with a full body warm-up and stretch.

WARM-UP

There are several ways to begin to warm the body before beginning a full stretching routine. You can march in place for five minutes. Some may prefer to do jumping jacks. Jumping jacks are best performed, by extending an alternating leg during every other jump. This allows each leg to receive an individual warm up symmetrically. For example, do one jumping jack in the regular fashion, then on the next jump, extend the right leg to the side an tap the heel to the ground. Follow this with another regular jumping jack, then extend the left leg to the side and tap the heel to the ground, and continue. A skips for five minutes are another great warm up. An A skip is skipping in place with exaggerated knee lifts.

ULTIMATE STRETCHING

Dynamic stretching is the form of stretching that I prefer. Dynamic stretching utilizes movement and momentum to propel the muscle into an extended range of motion. This form of stretching prepares the body for physical exertion and performance. Dynamic stretching increases the range of body movement, as well as increasing the blood and oxygen flow to soft tissues prior to physical exertion.

Note that all the stretches begin in the standing position, referred to as the *winning posture position.* Winning posture means that the body is completely erect, as if a string were pulling from the top of the head, shoulders back, back straight and stomach pulled in.

So, let's start stretching!

FIVE
ULTIMATE
TRANSFORMATIONS
STRETCHES

STRETCH #1 – KNEE TO CHEST

1. Stand tall with winning posture.

2. Raise and bend right leg, grab right leg just below the knee and pull knee to your chest. Lower right leg to floor.

3. Repeat this movement with the left leg. Repeat the sequence five times.

STRETCH #1 – KNEE TO CHEST

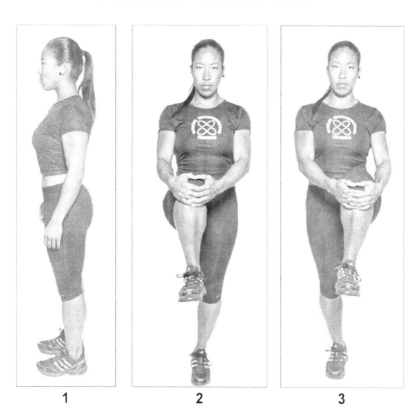

1   2   3

STRETCH #2 – REVERSE LUNGE

1.   Stand tall with winning posture. Keep the back straight and step forward with the right foot, approximately two feet.

2.   Lower hips, stretching the hip flexor of the right leg and the gluteus of left leg.

3.   Spring back to the starting position and repeat with left leg. Repeat the sequence five times.

STRETCH #2 – REVERSE LUNGE

1

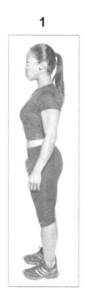

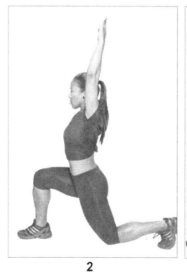

2

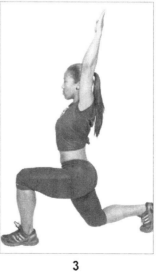

3

STRETCH #3 – HIP LIFTS

1. Stand tall with winning posture.

2. Raise the right foot towards the middle of the body. Grab the ankle of the right foot with the left hand. Grab the right knee with the right hand. With both hands, gently lift and pull the leg upward stretching the hip.

3. Lower the leg and repeat the motion with the left leg. Repeat the sequence five times.

STRETCH #3 – HIP LIFTS

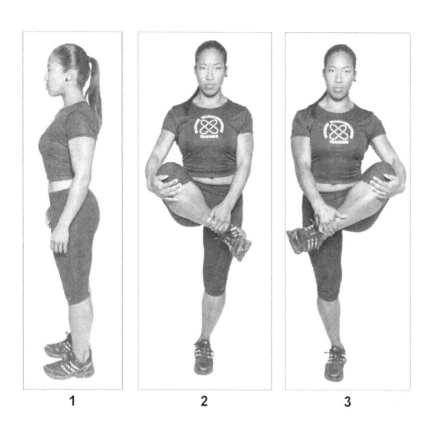

1   2   3

STRETCH #4 – QUAD STRETCH

1. Stand tall with winning posture.

2. Raise the right foot, reaching it toward the gluteus. Grab the foot with the right hand and pull the heel of the foot to the buttocks. Stand tall.

3. Lower the foot to the floor and repeat the motion with the left foot. Repeat the sequence five times.

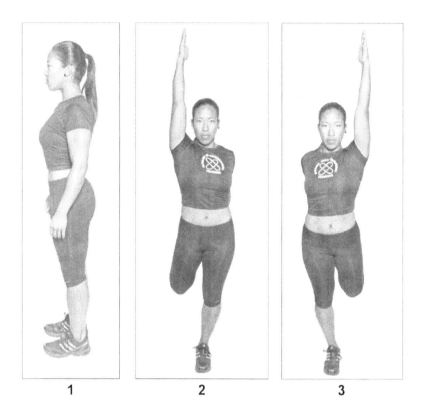

1   2   3

STRETCH #4 SIDE VIEW – QUAD STRETCH

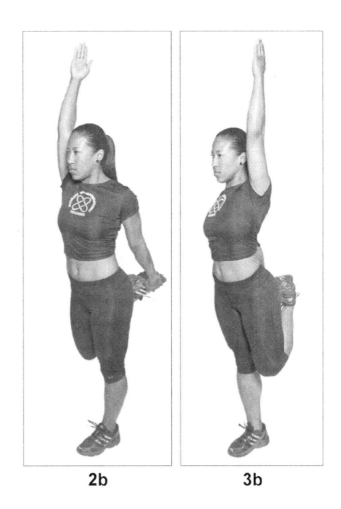

2b   **3b**

STRETCH #5 – STRAIGHT LEG KICK

1. Stand tall with winning posture.

2. Swing the right leg with a forward kick, extending the leg, keeping the right foot flexed and the leg straight. Extend the left arm toward the raised foot, slightly turning the torso toward the extended leg.

3. Lower the foot to the floor and repeat with the left leg. Repeat the sequence five times.

STRETCH #5 – STRAIGHT LEG KICK

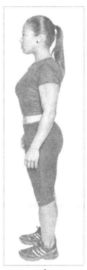

1

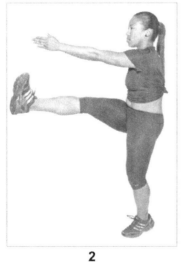

2

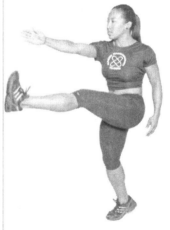

3

THREE BASIC WORKOUT PROGRAMS FOR TRANSFORMATION

PROGRAM

1

UTT WALKING – THE ULTIMATE PROGRAM

Walking is a gentle, low-impact exercise that can ease you into a higher level of fitness and health. Walking is one of your body's most natural forms of exercise. It is safe, simple and does not require practice, and the health benefits are numerous.

Before beginning any exercise program, particularly walking, you must first have the proper equipment for the task. While the list of equipment is minimal, it is very important to obtain a proper walking or running shoe. A running shoe is preferable over a walking shoe, because it has been made to absorb the shock and pounding that the body will incur during running. If you are over weight or a novice, the running shoe will help you prevent injury and trauma to your joints, until the body becomes accustomed to the exercise program.

Are your running shoes up to the task? Here is an easy way to find the answer: if you have a running shoe for a while and you want to know if the shoe is still good, i.e. shock absorbing, take the shoe in both hands and bend it to touch the toe to the heel. If the shoe shows resistance, it is still good. If the shoe touches easily, then it is time for another pair.

At the onset of a workout program, a proper shoe is a necessity and is the most important piece of equipment. It is also helpful for you to obtain a stop-watch, or a watch that keeps accurate time.

UTT WALKING PROGRAM

1. Determine the course that you will walk, i.e. the park in your neighborhood, at the beach, etc.

2. Warm-up with a 2 to 3 minute walk in place or slow walk. Then proceed with some light stretching.

3. Begin your walk at a gradual pace focusing on the process. That means to bend the arms at a 90-degree angle and walk with a foot strike that is heel to toe. Keep our abdomen contracted with your chest up. Think of the arms as your legs. If you want to increase or decrease your walking tempo, achieve this by increasing the speed of your arm swing, or by slowing your arm swing.

4. If the goal of walking for the day is 30 minutes, then your "actual" start time will commence after the first five minutes of the walk. The first five minutes will serve as your warm up. The body will then be ready to go!

5. Be mindful of your breathing. Inhale through your nose and exhale out of your mouth. If at anytime during the walk, you feel light headed or nauseous, slow down your pace and focus on controlling your breathing.

6. Time is the parameter by which you want to initially gage your walk. To receive increased

results begin to increase your walk time by 10 minutes every six walking days until you reach an hour of walking time. Upon reaching an hour of walking time, begin to focus on increasing the walking pace. Increase your pace to your fastest pace for one-to three-minute intervals and then settle back into a more comfortable pace for a five to seven-minute interval. As your body becomes comfortable with this type of training, you may be able to introduce running into your fitness plan.

Consistency in the workout is mandatory, once you have made the choice to make health and wellness a priority. Remember, make NO EXCUSES. Always maintain the thought that you can always make time to get a workout during the day, no matter what the circumstances.

PROGRAM

2

TRANSFORMATION 'TO GO' (40 REP) 6 EXERCISES

The Transformation to go program consists of a 40 Rep Workout that can be performed anywhere; next to the bed, at the park, the gym, or in a hotel. All that is required is your commitment! The 40 Rep workout is so named, because **every exercise will be completed in 4 sets of 10 repetitions (reps)**.

While four sets of each exercise is required, the beginning fitness level of an individual will ultimately determine the number of repetitions that may be accomplished at the start of the fitness journey. For example, one may complete four sets of five reps, or four sets of 25 reps, for each of the six exercises that follow. However, make sure you complete four sets with the number of repetitions that is comfortable for your fitness level.

EXERCISE ONE – SQUAT

The squat is a great exercise for developing the hip joint, gluteus maximus, quadriceps, hamstrings and lower back. (i.e., improves the look and function of the butt and hips).

EXECUTION

1. Start position: Stand tall with feet a little outside of shoulder width. Point toes slightly outside of the heels of the feet. Have arms straight and directly out in front of the body.

2. Pick a spot on the ceiling and while looking slightly up at the spot, lower the hips by bending at the knee. Remember to make sure that heels of the feet keep contact with the ground. Keep the head up and spine arched, and continue to focus on the spot on the ceiling.

3. After lowering the hips to a 100-degree angle, return to the standing position, by pushing off the heels of the feet. Extend fully to the standing position, with the spine arched and hips controlled. Keep the knees directly over the feet. The vertical position is reached once the hips complete the upward movement, thus, preventing hyper-extension of the knee joint.

EXERCISE ONE – SQUAT

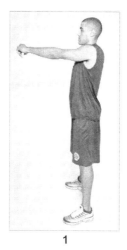

1

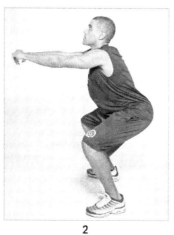

2

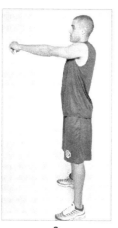

3

EXERCISE TWO – DEAD LIFT

The dead lift provides focused development of the lower back, with an emphasis on the hamstrings (i.e., strengthens and tones the back of the thigh and lower back).

EXECUTION

1. Start position: Stand tall with your feet set hip width apart, legs in a fixed position. The knees should not be "locked" in position. Shoulders should be back with a slightly arched back. The weight of the body is on the back half of the feet.

2. Shift the hips back and lower the hands toward the feet, while bending at the hips. Maintain a straight back. While lowering the upper body, the chin remains up and the shoulders remain back.

3. Activate the hamstrings and gluteus while returning to an upright position. Focus on pushing the hips back while maintaining a straight back.

EXERCISE TWO – DEAD LIFT

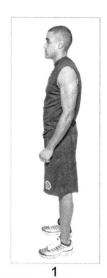

1

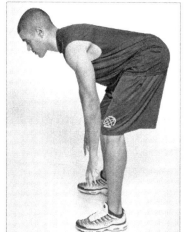

2

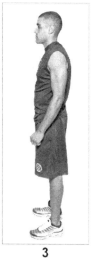

3

Exercise Three – Side Bend

This move focuses on core strength and flexibility. The side bend places an emphasis on internal and external obliques and deltoids (shoulders) (i.e., firms shoulders and stream-lines waist).

Execution

1. Start position: Stand upright with feet outside shoulder width. Keep a relaxed curve in the lower back and a slight bend in your knees. Bend both arms at the elbows, with hands even with the ears. Palms of both hands are facing the ceiling.

2. Bend at the waist, directly to the right side. At the same time, raise the opposite arm (left) up the right side of the body into the air and above the head, to full extension. The right arm remains pointing straight toward the ground. Bend back to the starting position.

3. Repeat the movement to the opposite side, bending to the left side, with the right arm extending up and over the head. One full repetition consists of a side bend to both sides of the body.

EXERCISE THREE – SIDE BEND

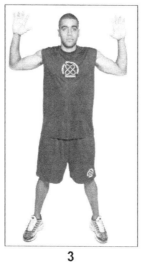

3

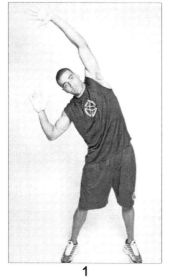

1

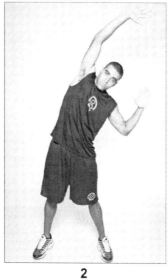

2

EXERCISE FOUR – BICEP CURL

The bicep curl focuses on arm strength with an emphasis on the front of the upper arm (bicep) (i.e., creates strong and toned upper arms).

EXECUTION

1. Start position: Stand upright, chest up with a slight curve in the lower back. Place arms to the side. With hands palm-side forward, make a fist.

2. Contract muscle in the arms, particularly the bicep. Curl the fist up toward the shoulder.

3. Relax and lower fist to starting position. Contract arm and repeat curl of fist to the shoulder

(As your fitness level increases, you may add weights or resistance bands. – **UTT Ready Pack**)

EXERCISE FOUR – BICEP CURL

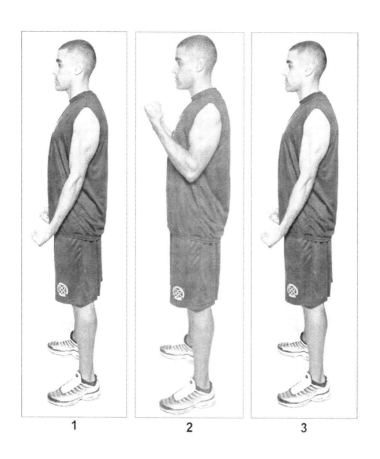

1 2 3

EXERCISE FIVE A – BEGINNING PUSH-UPS

Beginning push-ups develop overall upper body strength, core function, arms, chest and back. The development emphasis will be on the triceps and chest (i.e., lifts and tones arms, back and chest).

EXECUTION

1. Start position: Lay face down on the floor with the palm of the hands firmly placed just slightly outside the shoulders. Spread fingers to distribute weight and energy on the floor. Spread legs slightly, with toes and knees remaining on the floor. Keep hands even with solders and push the upper body upward until arms are vertically straight.

2. Lower the body to the floor and do not allow the chest come in contact with the floor.

3. Keep hands even with solders and push the upper body upward until arms are vertically straight. Remember to keep your back straight and control the upper body by keeping the abdominal muscles contracted. Repeat.

EXERCISE FIVE A – BEGINNING PUSH-UPS

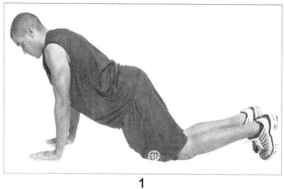

1

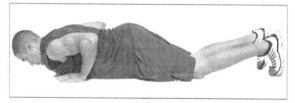

2

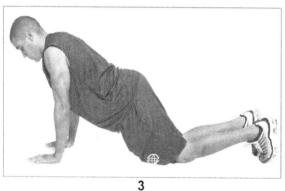

3

EXERCISE FIVE B – REGULAR PUSH-UPS

Regular push-ups are executed the same way, *except*, only the hands and toes are in contact with the floor (not the knees), through-out the entire exercise.

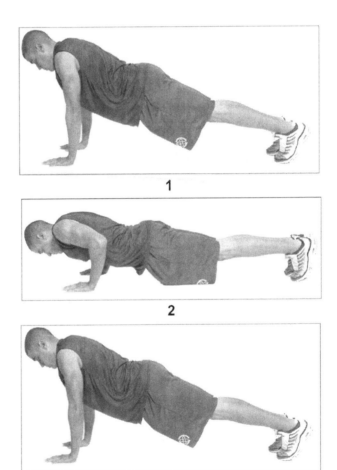

1

2

3

EXERCISE SIX – VACUUM CRUNCH

The vacuum crunch develops the upper and lower abdomen (i.e., flattens and strengthens the stomach muscles).

EXECUTION

Start position: Lay with the back on the ground and knees bent. Feet should be firmly planted on the floor. Cross arms across the chest, hugging the shoulders. This position prevents the chin from touching the chest.

Contract the abdomen and lift the shoulders from the floor, then roll the shoulders toward the bent knees. Focus on keeping the chin up. Make sure the hips remain in contact with the floor. Release the contraction and roll the back down to the floor. Repeat the exercise.

EXERCISE SIX – VACUUM CRUNCH

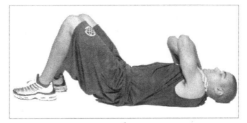

1

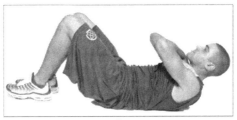

2

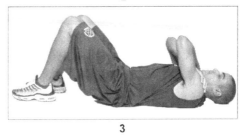

3

PROGRAM

3

BURPEE WORKOUT

The burpee workout is for the individual that is looking for an intermediate to advanced level workout. Burpees are a low impact, yet overall body, workout that incorporates components of strength, endurance and cardiovascular conditioning (i.e., full-body conditioning).

Burpees can be performed within the home, in the park, or in the gym. Just like the previous exercises, there is no special equipment required. Core strength will be vastly improved with continued incorporation of this workout.

The novice should begin with four sets of this exercise, while the more advanced may begin with 10 sets. Perform the exercise in increments of 5, 10, 15, 20 or 25 repetitions, again, based on your fitness level.

EXECUTION

1. Start position: Stand upright with enough room in front and behind to execute a regular push up.

2. From the start position, bend at the waist until you can place both hands on the floor and have a slight knee bend.

3. From this position, jump the feet back into a platform/plank position (same as regular pushup position).

4. Lower to the ground to initiate a regular push up.

5. Execute a full push up.

6. With hands remaining on the floor, jump to a bent knee position.

7. Finally, return to the start position.
(This will complete one full repetition.)

Take a timed rest of 30 to 90 seconds between sets, then repeat the exercise.

BURPEE

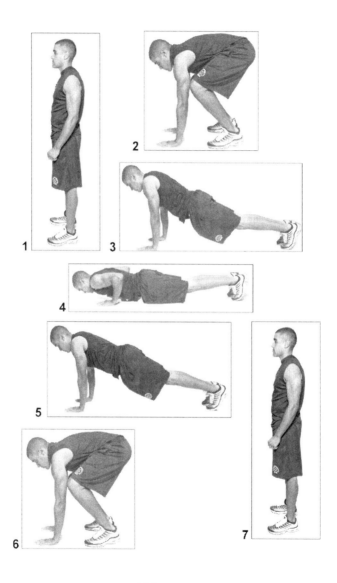

ENJOY THE BENEFIT
AND THE REWARD OF YOUR ENDURANCE

CHAPTER 11

YOUR ULTIMATE NEW LIFESTYLE – DAY 21

Look in the mirror. Yes, that's you! You look great, you feel great and you are expecting even greater things to come.

Everything in your world is changing for the better; your family, community and the world. You live in a state of peace, harmony, perfect health, wealth and prosperity. Your relationships are stronger and you feel a tremendous love from all the people that surround you. The possibilities for your personal life are unlimited. Nothing is out of reach. Your mental, physical and spiritual health is perfect, and you are in control! IT FEELS GOOD!!!!

All of a sudden, have you become lucky? Has God decided it is your turn to become prosperous? Have you found the perfect magic tonic that heals all ailments? No. All of these wonderful occurrences are happening because you have decided to change the negative thoughts of yourself and your surroundings to those that are more positive. The new positive thoughts have become deeply ingrained in your subconscious mind and you have formed new beliefs. This belief in good and unlimited potential, and your ability to think and do for yourself, has helped you recognize that you have a tremendous power. This infinite power has always been inside you. You are now using this power to make choices in every moment of your existence, here on earth. And "luck" has become your reality!

Now that you have begun to create a new YOU, repeat the exercise from chapter one. Note the changes and briefly explain to yourself what is causing the changes in the image that you previously had about yourself. This is a private and personal assessment to be evaluated only by the master of your discovery – YOU!

PICTURE OF SELF – SNAPSHOT #2

DATE: _____

HOW DO I FEEL ABOUT MYSELF TODAY?

MENTALLY? _____

_____

_____

_____

PHYSICALLY? _____

_____

_____

_____

SPIRITUALLY? _____

_____

_____

_____

WHERE DO I SEE MYSELF IN THE NEXT 12 MONTHS?

_____

_____

_____

WHERE DO I SEE MYSELF IN THE NEXT 24 MONTHS?

_____

_____

_____

WHERE DO I SEE MYSELF IN THE NEXT 5 YEARS?

_____

_____

_____

AM I CHOOSING TO CONTINUE TO DO THE WORK TO CHANGE?

[ ]YES, BECAUSE _____

_____

_____

COMPARE SNAPSHOT #2 WITH SNAPSHOT #1. NOTE
THE DIFFERENCES:

_____

_____

_____

_____

Continue to grow and know that every occurrence in your life presents opportunities for you to experience good (that which you are). Know that anything that you choose, when you fully <u>commit</u> with total <u>belief</u>, and give consistent <u>effort</u> without excuses, you will accomplish. Celebrate personal gratification through achievement. Your <u>confidence</u> to choose greater things is now commonplace. This is your everyday life. You are a master of your world. You have become a positive source of energy to your family, community and the world. Your energy duplicates itself in everything that surrounds you. This is Ultimate Health and Wellness. This is YOU, and this is your new evolving life.

I thank you for making a positive choice, and congratulate you on your current and future contributions. Your positive contributions improve your family. Your improving family strengthens the community. As communities improve across the planet, the world becomes a better place for us all.

Peace and be more!

BIO

Erich C. Nall is Owner and Founder of Ultimate Transformations Training in Los Angeles.

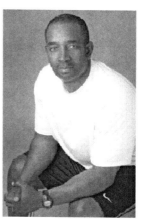

Erich, known fondly as Coach E, has been a prominent figure in the Los Angeles community throughout his life as an educator and promoter of health, physical fitness and self-improvement.

He has coached and trained many successful professional athletes, actors, models and others in the entertainment industry for over 18 years. Erich is a passionate <u>motivational speaker</u> and a dedicated life coach.

Erich is a frequent guest host on KJLH, 102.3 FM. He is a contributing writer of a weekly column in <u>Our Weekly Los Angeles</u> as well as a contributor to <u>Volleyball Magazine,</u> and The Los Angeles Sentinel. He is both a certified trainer and nutritionist who has spent the last 25 years learning from the best in sports training and conditioning. Erich holds his BA and MBA in Business and Economics.

"I want every individual to fall in love with the highest image of themselves." - *Coach E*

Erich is also the President and Founder of *Colle-*

giate Search Youth Organization, which offers tutorial support and academic assistance to students in the successful matriculation from elementary school through college graduation.

He lives in Los Angeles with his wife and three daughters.

To learn more about Ultimate Transformations Training, visit our Website at:

www.ultimatetransformations.com

Order 24 hours a day securely online.

TAKAMA Publishing House
14752 Crenshaw Blvd. Ste. 350
Gardena, California 90249

E-mail: info@ultimatetransformations.com

Breinigsville, PA USA
18 February 2011
255849BV00003B/1/P